DOES MY FATHER KNOW I'M HURT?

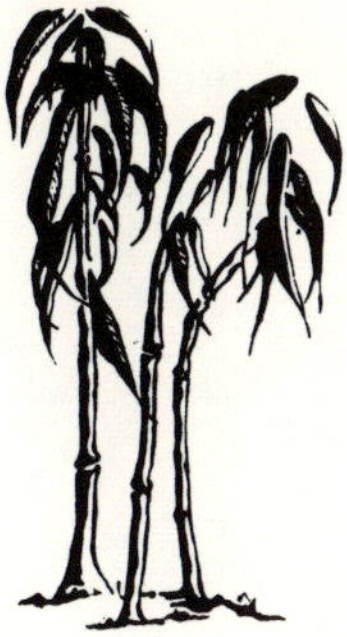

DOES MY FATHER KNOW I'M HURT?

David John Seel, M.D., F.A.C.S.

Illustrated by Peggy Bradford Long

TYNDALE HOUSE PUBLISHERS
Wheaton, Illinois

Coverdale House Publishers Ltd., London, England

Library of Congress Catalog Card No. 70-155975

SBN 8423-0670-6, paper SBN 8423-0671-4, cloth

First printing April, 1971

Printed in United States of America

Contents

Illustrations

Introduction

This is a remarkable book, telling the stories of individuals whose lives were blighted by cancer and of the loving ministry of a Christian physician combined with the highest degree of modern professional skill on their behalf — all told in remarkably beautiful prose.

The author has had exceptional training in his field of cancer research, in his surgical skills, and in modern techniques with X ray, cobalt, and other curative or palliative measures.

But he has more than that — a deep personal experience with Christ the Great Physician, a personality which radiates love for God and men, and rare carefulness and perseverance in carrying out the necessary steps for the welfare of his patients.

Beyond this, Dr. Seel has a gift of expression which makes this book a delight to read and which takes the reader along with him into a physician-patient relationship that sees the pathetic need for compassion and skillful treatment fulfilled by more than physical restoration — the presence and power of the living Christ.

Dr. Seel's professional qualifications are of the highest. A graduate of Tulane University (Phi Beta Kappa) and of Tulane Medical School, he has done graduate work at Charity Hospital in New Orleans, Memorial Hospital for cancer and allied diseases in New York, and is a Diplomate of the American Board of Surgery, a Fellow of the Society of Head and Neck Surgeons, a Fellow of the American College of Surgeons, a Member of the James Ewing Society and of many other learned and technical organizations. He is also the author of numerous scientific papers in leading surgical journals.

He is Chief of Oncological Surgery at the Presbyterian Medical Center in Chonju, Korea, and Director of that institution. He is also Associate Clinical Professor of Surgery at Yonsei University in Seoul, as well as Consultant in Surgery for the Korean Army.

L. Nelson Bell, M.D., F.A.C.S.

Preface

For one whose work is primarily concerned with the treatment of patients with cancer, the question posed by Richard Kim in his novel *The Martyred* was particularly poignant: "Your God — is he aware of the suffering of his people?"[1] The question arose out of the horror, destruction, and misery of the Korean conflict of 1950-1953. The question remains relevant in the face of the disasters which continue to beset human existence. These disasters are sometimes collective but in the final analysis are always individual.

The setting for the experiences upon which this presentation is based is Presbyterian Medical Center, better known in Korea as "Jesus Hospital," in the city of Chonju. It is now inaccurate to say that this is a mission hospital. It is rather a witnessing medical community of international character, transcultural in orientation, its participants bound together in a common allegiance to Jesus Christ. Out of deference for the theme which I have chosen, I must omit a description of the life and work of this institution and of the team which labors there, but it is not out of a lack of appreciation for colleagues whose dedication has inspired me. In particular I must express my gratitude to Dr. Paul Crane, whose vision set the ship's course, and who was the instrument for my calling to this work; to Miss Margaret Pritchard, R.N., elder statesman and balance wheel for the crew; and for the memory of Dr. Frank Keller, who gave his life for the dream.

But this is not primarily a mission book. It is rather an effort to answer honestly the question posed by Richard Kim in the context of the cancer struggle in Korea. It is hoped that this may help some who at times have felt bewildered by the enigma of tragic destiny to find some meaning to their grief or despair. It is also suggested that every Christian has a role in the answer.

I am indebted to Dr. Kyoung-jik Han, of the Young Nak Presbyterian Church, for the Bruised Reed concept.

This book would not have been written without the faith and the encouragement of Mary, my wife, whose love has never failed me.

1

"Anyone to save it. Anyone who wants it. If there's none I'm sunk. We all are. Doomed. Damned."[2]

"Fear not, for I have redeemed you. I have called you by name, you are mine. When you pass through the waters I will be with you; and through the rivers, they shall not overwhelm you; when you walk through fire you shall not be burned, and the flame shall not consume you. For I am the Lord your God, the Holy One of Israel, your Savior. . . . You are precious in my eyes, and honored, and I love you."[3]

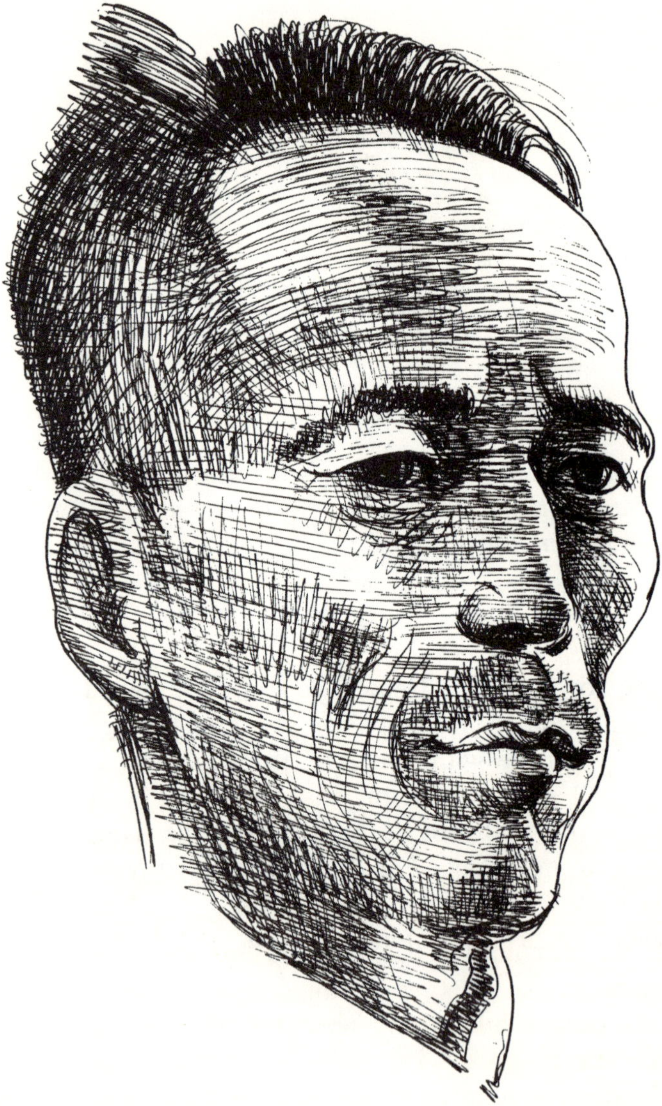

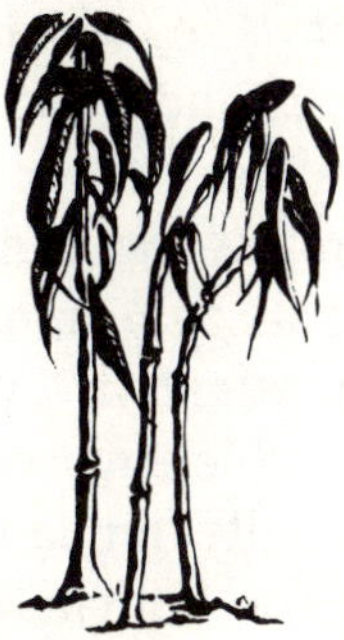

THE BRUISED REED

Southward from the Diamond Mountains above the demilitarized zone, along the eastern shore of the peninsula, the Great White Range dominates the terrain of Korea. Below the 38th Parallel it gives off a series of branches that run southwest toward the Yellow Sea, leaving scarcely a third of the land flat enough for cultivation. But near the western coast there appear occasionally flat expanses of land between the mountainous fingers. Here the rice fields extend as far as the eye can see, to horizons broken by distant hills rising abruptly like islands above the sea of grain. The fields are crisscrossed by an elaborate system of canals and dikes, so that even the villages are laid out in rectangular fashion to conform to the geometry of irrigation.

The southern bank of the Manggyong estuary ends in a tongue of land which juts out into the tidal mud-flats. Near land's-end lies the village of Changja-Ri, a hamlet of fifty or sixty thatch-roofed houses. One of them, at the bamboo-clogged dike's edge, while differing in only minor degree from the rest, reveals to the attentive eye the marks of a progressive farmer: chickens cooped rather than running free; a carefully tended vegetable garden; and a compost pile for human refuse. This is the home of Byong-Ho Choi.

He is known throughout the township of Kwang-whal as the man who for seventeen years bore the stigma of death.

Late in July 1950, soldiers of the People's Army arrived in Changja-Ri and took positions on the hilltop at land's-end overlooking the sea. Shortly a delegation came to Choi's home and arrested him for being the village chief. He was taken to the county seat of Kimje and beaten with canes until his scalp was a pulp and his back sliced and his left shoulder blade fractured and exposed. The wounds festered in prison so he was released after a time, but the shoulder ulcer never healed in spite of the efforts of several years and eventually the chronic draining pus exerted a carcinogenic effect.

When he ultimately came to the Presbyterian Medical Center after seventeen years, the stigma had become a cancer, the legacy of hate become the mark of death, as large as one of his hands, foul and draining. And in coming, he became part of the procession of misery that silently congregates from terraced hillsides, from valley hamlets, from a thousand coastal islands, from river bed shanties, from market sheds, caves, and hovels — all stigmatized by the same infernal death-process eroding in the centercore of physical life. Frail as the bamboo shoots growing in the canal by his home, Choi had been trampled as if some wild animal had thrashed among the reeds, and was now become symbolic of his nation and his people, bruised at midstalk, a constant reminder of the frailty of human expectations in a century of greed and strife. That bruise had become self-perpetuating and inexorable; for the external bootprint of the aggressor had now begotten a treason within his very fibers.

Byong-Ho Choi's first clinic visit was thus the end of a pilgrimage. He came as would a prisoner to the court of last resort, pleading his life. He joined the throng waiting for hope in the corridors of a mission hospital; and when his biopsy confirmed the diagnosis his name was added to the Cancer Registry to join those of his fellow victims. Yet he was more fortunate than the majority of cancer patients: his lesion was technically resectable, though he lost most of his shoulder blade.

Today he stands erect in his village, laboring with his fellows at planting and at harvest, free at last of his despicable wound. The bruised reed is restored to wave its fronds among the bamboo trees.

Mr. Choi's story has a symbolic dimension. This book is concerned with men who have come under a curse which jeopardizes their existence. A humble person in a disadvantaged environment attacked by malignant forces: these are the ingredients of helplessness and defeat. To some extent this may serve as a capsule of the human predicament.

Our pragmatic world rejects sentimental ideals. Transcendent visions will soon be tested in the grime of life, and the noble will be discarded with the spurious unless it is relevant to the realities of human existence. The cancer patient is not unique in his experience of suffering, and there undoubtedly have been more brutal, more agonizing experiences in the annals of men. The anguish of the people of Viet Nam cannot be lightly dismissed. It would be pretentious to attempt to ascribe meaning to the meaningless destruction of modern war. It would be presumptuous to claim any new comprehension of the chaos which has engulfed individuals caught in the cross fire of ideological struggle. We may only speak of what we know. I can identify with the silent horror of the cancer victim. I can, if only briefly, feel the unrelenting stabbing headache of the man whose growth has eroded the skull base. I can understand the disgust toward oneself felt by the patient whose rotting tumor fills the room with stench. For a few moments I can wear the skin of the victim dying with nausea, robbed of dignity, his disfigurement an affront and an embarrassment to his loved ones. I know what it means to die of shame. The human spirit in extremis rises from the pit to hurl the question, *"Is God aware of the sufferings of his people?"*

The answers which will be proposed to this question presuppose the validity of spiritual values, and of faith in the affirmation of those values. This is not a scientific treatise. It does nevertheless inquire into ultimate truth: Is there a basis for believing in a compassionate God? Does suffering have significance for life? Is participation in suffering then normative for man in God's plan for redemption? How does the human spirit in distress experience God's covenant of mercy? If in the experience of the cancer patient it can ever be found that curse was translated into blessing, death into life, stigma into salvation, and despair into hope, the testimony concerning what brought this about has universal significance for mankind in trouble.

In this chapter, and the next, we will consider the first of these questions, that of the existence of a compassionate God in his awareness of stricken humanity. What does he say? What does he do? What is the nature of the human wound, and how may it be healed?

* * *

In the sixth and seventh centuries B.C. there occurred an outpouring of wisdom from China, India, and the Middle East. Confucius called for benevolence and loyalty as foundations of the virtuous state. Gautama began his teaching of the noble eight-fold path of enlightenment. And Isaiah set down the concept of the Suffering Servant. Confucius sought virtue in harmony with the will of heaven, but never acknowledged a personal God. Gautama sought escape from the misery of existence, but also withheld recognition of a Divine Being. Isaiah claimed to speak for Jehovah, the Lord God of Israel, when he wrote:

> Behold my servant, whom I uphold,
> my chosen, in whom my soul delights;
> I have put my Spirit upon him,
> he will bring forth justice to the nations.
> He will not cry nor lift up his voice,
> or make it heard in the street;
> A bruised reed he will not break,
> and a dimly burning wick he will not quench.
> He will faithfully bring forth justice.
> He will not fail or be discouraged
> till he has established justice in the earth;
> and the coastlands wait for his law.[4]

The prophecy might have remained but a dream, the vision of a man of faith. His words might have been lost or buried in some urn in a Dead Sea cave. Yet the concept of a Suffering Servant who did not lift up his voice, of a chosen one who would not be discouraged by the bruised reeds and smoldering wicks of the human race — this concept survived; and when a carpenter's son walked through Palestine not only proclaiming the righteousness of God, but also "moved with compassion" in his quiet procession between sickness and anguish, some there were who saw in him the "Spirit of the Lord." Indeed, this Jesus, identifying himself with the prophetic utterance of Isaiah, chose as his manifesto the Scripture,

> The Spirit of the Lord is upon me,
> Because he has anointed me to preach good
> tidings to the afflicted,
> He has sent me to bind up the brokenhearted,
> To proclaim liberty to the captives
> and the opening of prison to those who
> are bound;
> To proclaim the year of the Lord's favor.[5]

It remained for him to be sacrificed by the political and religious leaders of his day, yet never has a man so lived, never has a man so died. Those who beheld his glory testified that it was that of the only Son of the Father, that indeed God had visited this planet, sharing the flesh and blood of his human creatures, partaking of their very nature, identifying with them to the point of death, indeed tasting that death for every man so that God might liberate all those who through fear of death have been subject to lifelong bondage.

Life is frail. Those of us who attend it in its

more fragile moments know well the susceptibility of the human organism to injury, infection, degeneration, and decay. But far deeper than physical afflictions are those which attack the human spirit. No assault is more brutal than that which casts aside an individual as beneath concern. In the survival economy of the East, human life is often considered a commodity not worth setting on the balance. Why the effort to save a beggar's life? Why subject a family (for there are no individuals) to the expense and risk of a surgical procedure? Why prolong life if a man may not again earn the food he will consume? If the Korean is prone to look upon the dark side of the coin, it must be remembered that centuries of disaster have prepared him to surrender to death rather than struggle against odds. When he figuratively bares his chest before the physician, crying, "Give me to live!", the poignancy of his plea is that of a man under sentence, a life swinging like a pendulum between fond hope and utter despair.

The bruise may not be visible. Evidently the outcasts, the downtrodden, the afflicted, and the forgotten qualify as the products of a callous society. When Christ summoned the weary and heavy laden, he also meant those burdened with guilt. Just as fungi, bacteria, and insect parasites may attack the roots and stems of plants, so also the germ of sin may corrode the stalk from within, interrupting the flow of life from the root and causing graceful fronds to wither and die. Sin bruises the human spirit at the core. In the clinical sphere, an externally visible tumor mass immediately challenges the surgeon to an effort in its extirpation. Yet removal of the tumor is futile in the presence of untreated septicemia, futile when a rampant infection spreads through the blood to every organ of the body. Sin threatens life as does overwhelming sepsis, poisoning the total personality. And it is in the total blackness of pervasive guilt that we hear the news of hope:

> The bruised reed he will not break,
> and a dimly burning wick he will not quench.
> He will not fail or be discouraged. . . .

For the Lord knows our condition. He also grew up like a tender plant, and like a root out of dry ground. He came forth as a shoot from the stump of Jesse, and the branch that grew from those roots is become the tree of life whose leaves are for the healing of the nations. He was bruised for our iniquities, upon him was the chastisement that made us whole, and with his stripes we have been healed.

How can the bruise of Christ heal the afflictions and infirmities of man? Is it reasonable to speak of being healed by his stripes?

A discussion of the psychology of guilt is beyond the scope of this book. It is evident, however, that the human conscience requires that the forgiveness of sin be costly, the cost proportionate to the guilt. Even between men, cheap forgiveness is meaningless. Guilt is not removed by the wave of God's hand, for that would be tantamount to saying, "Forget it, it doesn't make any difference." God is not worth worshiping unless he is holy, and therefore human sin does make a difference to him.

The dilemma of man burdened by guilt is precisely that he knows his guilt must be somehow expiated, atoned, made good — yet this is beyond his moral resources. It is in this situation that the chastisement of Christ in his stead provides the only solution. When a man's heart is flabby with disease and failing, he may, under certain circumstances, be considered as a candidate for heart transplantation. In this situation the life of the recipient is purchased at the cost of the remaining life of the donor, whose brain is already dead. The chastisement that makes us whole was also costly: our guilt was removed at the cost of the life of Christ. In either situation the recipient must give his consent, must make his own decision on the basis of a recognition of his own helplessness, and in faith that the life of the donor may heal him. The analogy is inescapable, for in God's operating room the offer is also contingent upon faith, "that whosoever believeth on him should not perish."[6]

This is the message entrusted to the church. If we can accept Christ's offer in faith God will not count our guilt, our corruption, our decay against us. The bruised reed he will not break, the wick encrusted with smut and grime he will not quench. Much rather in Christ he will heal, cleanse, restore; he will not fail or be discouraged until he has removed the curse at the cost of his cross. And in the proclamation of this message he gives to his disciples the power to transform the baneful and malevolent into blessing. Byong-Ho Choi was doubly cursed when he came to Jesus Hospital, and in the struggle to eradicate his cancer the deeper enemy was not ignored. Every confrontation with physical disease is at most a twilight reflection of the greater struggle, the outcome of which will be revealed in some distant dawn, a conflict in which God's encompassing mercy and holiness grapple with the defiant and malignant forces of evil over the destiny of every human soul. In the midst of the fray, all but overwhelmed by the contending spiritual worlds that envelop him, stands the individual, both victim and aggressor, slave to sin yet free to believe that the seeking, searching, yearning God did indeed taste death for every man, was indeed bruised for our iniquities, does indeed reach forth his hand of love to grasp him from the torment. To him Jesus addressed his promise, "I will not leave you desolate; I will come to you."[7]

The promise of Christ becomes the imperative of his disciples. Some have ministered to the untouchables, others to the proud; some to the disgraced, others to the ungrateful. My parish is an assembly of cancer victims in southwest Korea. This is my flock, this is my garden of trampled flowers and bruised reeds. I am grateful to them. From them I have learned the dimensions of courage and the cost of faith.

2

"Whether the disease is found to be curable or incurable, dealing with the patient who has cancer is a struggle with the idea of death and the process of dying. . . . The patient inherently feels helpless when confronted with the diagnosis of cancer, and unlike other diseases in his experience, he can exercise no control over it; the patient senses that nothing he does or refrains from doing can alter the course of the disease or the inevitable end."[8]

"For I know that my Redeemer liveth, and that he shall stand at the latter day upon the earth: and though after my skin worms destroy this body, yet in my flesh shall I see God."[9]

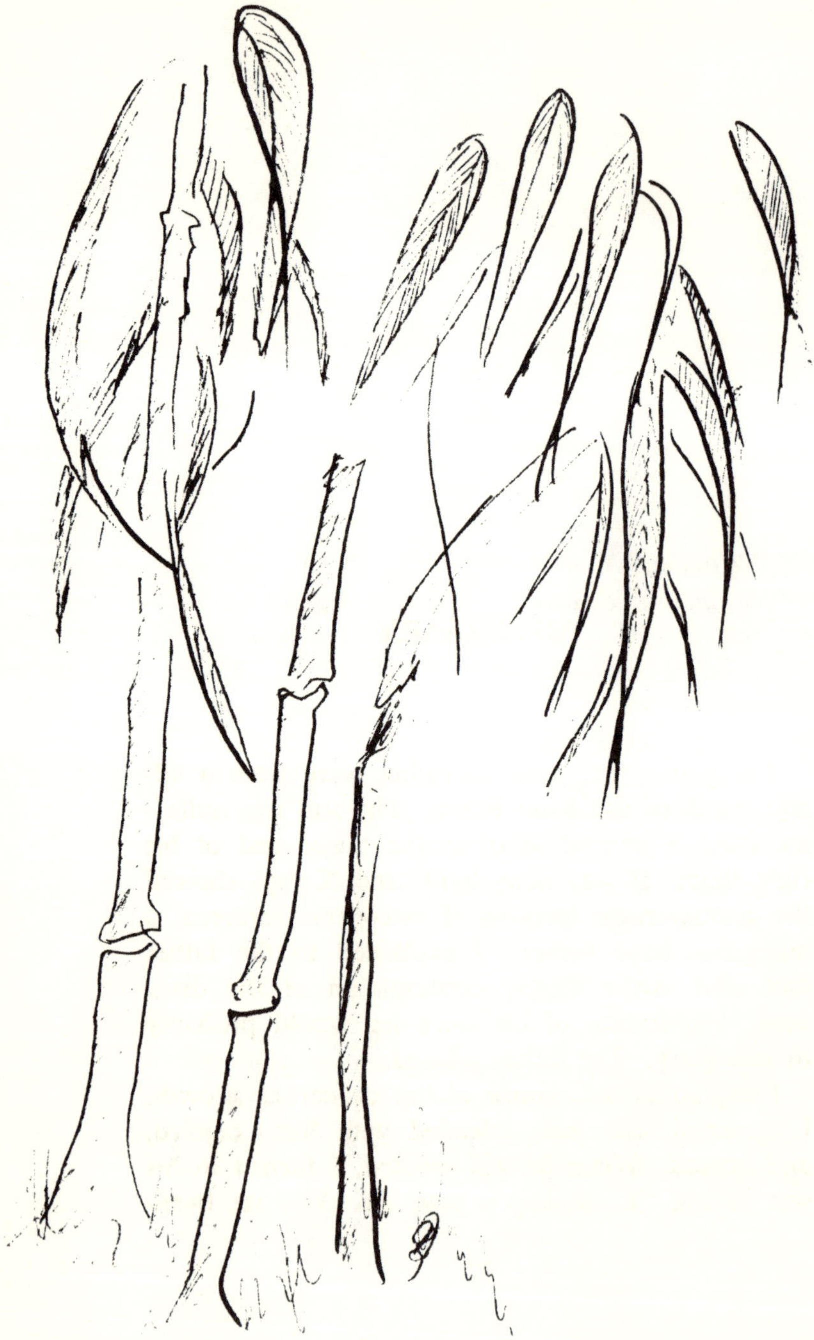

ADVERSARY

The young man and his father were from a village north of the Kum River. The son was suffering from a painful lump at the lower end of his right thigh. It was bony hard, and X rays showed the characteristic features of osteogenic sarcoma, a malignant bone tumor. I explained to the father that after tissue biopsy confirmation of the diagnosis, amputation of his son's leg would probably be necessary. The father refused.

I explained the nature of the cancerous growth, I reasoned with him, pleaded with him, cajoled, and argued. When he still refused, I turned to his son, saying, "Look, this is *your* life. You are twenty-three. Even though you lose your leg, you will be able to walk with an artificial limb. This is your only chance. Don't throw your life away!" The young man replied, "I would like to have surgery, but I must obey my father."

Finally, I asked our Korean medical colleagues to seek to persuade the old man to give his consent. They reported to me later that it was not a question of the hospital bill, nor did he disbelieve my warnings. It was simply a matter of face. The father could not permit the disgrace in his village of having an amputee for a son! And I thought to myself: which is the greater cancer, the malignant neoplasm in the boy's leg, or the one in his father's heart?

Cancer appears to be common among the Korean people. There are no valid national statistics to verify the experience at our own hospital, where approximately one of every twenty new patients — pregnant mothers, tuberculosis victims, parasite carriers, and malnourished infants all included — one of twenty has cancer.

(During the six-year period from January 1963 until December 1968 over 3,032 new primary lesions were discovered among 65,000 new patients. Since the latter figure includes new-born infants, which averaged 500 per year, the ratio of cancer diagnoses becomes approximately 3,000 of 62,000 new patients.)

The stomach is most commonly affected in men, followed by liver and lung cancer. In women, the uterine cervix ranks first, the stomach second, the breast third. The tragedy of cancer in an underdeveloped nation is that coping with it is so far beyond the means of the people and of the government that it is dismissed as a totally irrelevant matter. Industrialization, electric power, communications — these command the efforts of the bureaucrats. Sanitation, birth control, and communicable diseases absorb the energies of the health authorities. Perhaps this is as it should be. Perhaps it is proper that government should write off, as expendable, afflicted human life so that available food supplies and job opportunities should go further. But such calculated dispassion in the brokerage of human life suddenly becomes meaningless when the cancer is found in one's own bowels. Respect for the sanctity of life begins when a man considers that the next fellow wants to live, to fulfill his dreams, to build a home, to raise children, to "do his thing," as much as he does.

The tradition of tragedy may have made the Korean people callous to the sacredness of human existence. Yet I can testify that when the individual's life is on the block, his anxiety, his desperate hope, his fear and grief are no different from that of any other race, except in one respect: it involves the immediate family far more than it does in the West. It would appear that there are no individual decisions, only family decisions; and though this may surround the patient with comfort, it also makes a grim diagnosis the more grim, for the *family* must decide within the framework of its limited financial, moral, and spiritual resources.

There are no social agencies. The hospital will offer free care if convinced the family is making a sacrificial effort. But the pagan family may refuse to expend its resources for the life of one of its members. I can imagine fewer more poignant dramas than that in which a family group considers whether the life of a child, or the curing of a cancer of an aging father, is worth the cost of mortgaging the rice crop or of selling the family cloth. (Due to the instability of Korean currency in the past, the traditional scheme for family savings is to purchase a bolt of expensive material.) In the family council a "survival of the fittest" criterion will often determine the destiny of the afflicted member, for the individual has no intrinsic value in Oriental thought. It is the family which must be safeguarded in a society scrabbling for existence. This is the context of the cancer struggle in Korea.

My interest in oncology began in 1956 during my early years in Korea. The advanced tumor pathology which I encountered at Presbyterian Medical Center was startling and apalling, and led me to seek further training in this field. After completing a senior surgical residency at Memorial-Sloan Kettering Cancer Center in New York I returned to Korea, seeking to implement a more aggressive thrust in the management of cancer patients. A Tumor Clinic and Cancer Registry have been established. The patients who stream through the clinic on Wednesday — tumor day — are for the most part grateful patients, though many bear the marks of radiation therapy or the scars of surgical attack. Yet they are keenly aware of their hazardous fortune; they live on "the raw edge of a thin hope."[10]

It may seem surprising that a mission hospital would become involved in such an effort in the field of cancer control in an underdeveloped nation. We believe the endeavor to be appropriate, urgent, and expressive. It is *appropriate* precisely because the cancer patient lives in fear, and Christ died in order to set free those who live their whole lives a prey to the fear of death. It is *urgent* because in the cancer victim the life-death balance is geared to a time-clock, and the eternal destiny of a human soul becomes an issue which can no longer be avoided. It is *expressive* because the character of the struggle required to eradicate cancer illustrates both the compassion and tenacity of God's quest for man as do few other endeavors in the Kingdom enterprise.

This is not an individual undertaking. Medicine today is too complex, and our patient load too physically demanding, for one man. My colleagues include Paul Crane, K. Y. Lee, Dorothea Sich, David Chu, and Jehoom Yang. Our surgical mortality has been low, our five-year cure rates, in view of the advanced pathology we must cope with, satisfactory in comparison with data from medical centers in America. Only God knows how far the witness of this work may reach. It is our experience that a medical disciple of Christ who does not cringe from dressing the foul ulcer, who is not dismayed by advanced disease, who does not abandon his charge however hopeless, may also reach into his innermost soul.

Cancer is defined as a growth of new cells which proliferate without control and which serve no useful function. At some point in the normal regeneration of tissues one cell becomes abnormal: it reproduces at an increased rate, breaking loose from those factors within the body which regulate the growth of tissues. Its progeny are abnormal and each cell passes on to its daughter cells the same unrestrained growth potential which disregards the health of the body as a whole in its reckless multiplication.

The physician who would engage this enemy in combat must be aware of the nature of his antagonist. The first characteristic of cancer is *insidiousness*. Cancer gives no rattlesnake warning of its presence. Numerous "doublings" are required before the tumor reaches the minimal critical size required for detection. Since the growth rate is geometrical, that part of a tumor's life cycle which occurs prior to diagnosis (i.e., the pre-clinical phase) is generally far longer than the period between diagnosis and death in the untreated case. The race may be far spent before the physician, however alert, can throw his efforts into the struggle. Cancer may be thought of as a conspirator which lurks in the recesses of the human organism; too often the insurrection has gathered too much momentum when the plot is discovered.

A second feature of cancer is *autonomy.* Disregarding the normal limitations of growth, the cancer cells grow relentlessly, spreading near and far, penetrating vital tissues in a headlong uncontrolled proliferation which leads inevitably to the destruction of its host unless it is completely eradicated.

The last of the characteristics we must mention is *anaplasia,* or the loss of organization and useful function. Cancer is parasitic. The tumor cells serve no good purpose whatever. They obey their own laws of unbridled initiative at the expense of the well-being of the host.

In the struggle to overcome this devilish process the therapist must appropriate some of the relentlessness of his antagonist, constantly searching for disease, employing every weapon he can bring to bear upon it, ever seeking to improve his skill, continually reevaluating his policies, fighting into the black of night and sometimes until the fragile dawn of victory. He joins with the patient in a battle in which no quarter is given or asked, a battle which he may sometimes win, or sometimes lose, but which he never ceases fighting. His philosophy was expressed by the Welsh poet, Ethelwyn Wetherald:

> My orders are to fight;
> Then if I bleed, or fail,
> Or strongly win, what matters it?

God only doth prevail.
The servant craveth naught
Except to serve with might.
I was not told to win or lose, —
My orders are to fight.[11]

For the cancer surgeon the battle becomes an intensely personal conflict. In the operating room he spends hours attacking the malignant growth, dissecting, circumscribing, blocking spread here, sacrificing tissue there, assaulting this evil thing from every side, at all costs trying to avoid cutting through its invisible tentacles, lest tumor cells spill into the surgical field, defeating him from the goal of a lasting cure. It is often a tense, dramatic struggle. Obviously, distant spread indicates incurability, as does involvement of an organ which is vital. Yet in some situations the surgeon must commit himself to a hazardous procedure before the evidence of curative resectability is at hand. His options become problematical: whether to risk a life to save it before he is convinced the risk has curative purpose. The tension mounts, the pace intensifies, the surgical risks escalate, and the surgeon must now struggle not only against his implacable antagonist but also against his own fear that either the aggressiveness of his attack or, conversely, his hesitancy to press the assault may cost the life he is agonizing to save. Fencing on a tightrope, he pursues his quarry. On and on, deeper and deeper, higher and higher, until at last the tumor is out, the demon exorcised, the enemy conquered.

But the victory is elusive, and the chance of a cure problematical. The tenacity of the therapist and the rapport between physician and patient are essential ingredients for improving the measure of success which may be obtained. The medical disciple of Christ enters into a contract with his patient from which he is never released as long as his patient lives. He must continually exhort his patient to courage, can never be too weary to go one step further in pursuit of a greater margin of safety, and can never abandon him even though there be nothing left to offer him medically. Locked hand-in-hand in a common life-death battle they must fight on; and if the physician be called to walk with him into the valley of shadows, then walk he must, supporting the patient's faith, comforting his despair, holding before him the hope and the assurance of a new resurrection in Christ Jesus.

At Chonju we are anxious for our house staff to appropriate this concept of responsibility. However often the patient may fail to keep his end of the bargain, the doctor must track him down, hound him back to Tumor Clinic for reevaluation and therapy. A biopsy is more than just another test, for a positive biopsy is a death sentence for the patient if not acted upon. A radical cancer operation is more than a skillful surgical exercise; it is the patient's golden day, his own great opportunity to escape destruction. And Tumor Clinic is more than simply the follow-up of an interesting case: it is a time of hope or reckoning as the doctor scrutinizes his patient for that early recurrence he might yet cure.

Here the issues of life are laid bare. The Christian physician who assumed a trusteeship for his patient's physical life must also accept involvement in his spiritual fate. There is no room for false modesty or religious squeamishness. The patient has a right to the truth. He has placed his entire self in the physician's hands. Many of the patients are living on borrowed time while the clock of life ticks away its last days, and soon the opportunity for claiming Christ as Savior and Lord for the remission of sins will be lost, and the patient must face his Maker.

Faced with the critical issue of the eternal destiny of the human soul, the Christian physician knows well the impact of Paul's exclamation, "Woe is unto me if I preach not the gospel!"[12]

A cancer surgeon worthy of the term will develop a belligerent sense of outrage toward his enemy. Cancer has indeed come to signify to me the embodiment of evil, a prototype of Satan. Yet, by comparison, how feeble is our moral indignation toward our spiritual adversary? Is there a more vivid way to describe the work of Satan than by the characteristics of cancer? We described him a moment ago: insidious, relentless, parasitic, deceptive, totally self-centered, serving no useful function, rebelling against his protector. It is not difficult to see a parallel between the behavior of cancer in the human organism and the behavior of evil in the human soul:

> Their throat is an open sepulchre;
> with their tongues they have used deceit;
> the poison of asps is under their lips:
> Whose mouth is full of cursing and bitterness:
> Their feet are swift to shed blood;
> Destruction and misery are in their ways:
> And the way of peace have they not known:
> There is no fear of God before their eyes.[13]

The simile must be taken one step further. The power of evil unceasingly seeks to infiltrate into the body of Christ, the Church. Of each cell Christ requires total allegiance. An organ made of cells which are not functioning on behalf of the body's well-being is a sick organ. If we were to personalize each cell and attribute to it free will, we might say that a cell which is not committed to the health of the body is a pathologic cell. A cell is not responsible for the resources of life; that is the task of the Head of the body. For us, only to function. When we cease to function we are dead; when we reject our allegiance, when we refuse submission to the Head, when we rebel from our commitment, we are cancerous.

A man's ultimate allegiance determines his course. The Evil One adopts every guise of pleasure, power, and pride to subvert man's loyalty to God. Once caught in the vice of addiction, whether to heroin or to prejudice, whether to alcohol or to ambition, all too soon the captive may exercise no control over his cancer. He is helpless before the inevitable, enmeshed in a web-pattern from which there is no escape. He can no longer control his actions. What he would do he cannot; what he knows to be despicable is what he will do.

"O wretched man that I am! who shall deliver me from the body of this death?"[14] The despairing outburst of Paul is the cry of our century, never more human, never more poignant. Yet in the midst of the spiritual chaos of our age the Hound of Heaven stalks and pursues the possessed and the afflicted with relentless mercy, implacable compassion. One came and bore the impact of all of the cancers of the human race, of all the filth and hatred and corruption, and died horribly — died of cancer — only to rise triumphant over him who has the power of death, Satan our adversary. God's defeat became a victory; God's gallows became the banner of the redeemed!

The first reply to our inquiry has now been given.

It might perhaps have been questioned whether Jehovah, Lord of Hosts, could sympathize with the misery of Job. And if God's revelation had closed with the words of the prophets, we would yet be waiting for the vindication of his promise not to break the trampled weed, not to quench the sputtering wick, to feed his flock like a shepherd, to give power to the faint, to heal the people from their sorrows. But no longer. The God of compassion became flesh and shared in human suffering, was stricken, in fact, far beyond human capacity to suffer, in order that the curse upon man might be transformed into an eternal blessing.

3

"No man is an Iland, intire of it selfe; every man is a peece of the Continent, a part of the maine; if a Clod bee washed away by the Sea, Europe is the lesse, as well as if a Promontorie were, as well as if a Mannor of thy friends or of thine owne were; any man's death diminishes me, because I am involved in Mankinde; And therefore never send to know for whom the bell tolls; It tolls for thee."[15]

"For continually, while still alive, we are being surrendered into the hands of death, for Jesus' sake, so that the life of Jesus also may be revealed in this mortal body of ours. Thus death is at work in us, and life in you."[16]

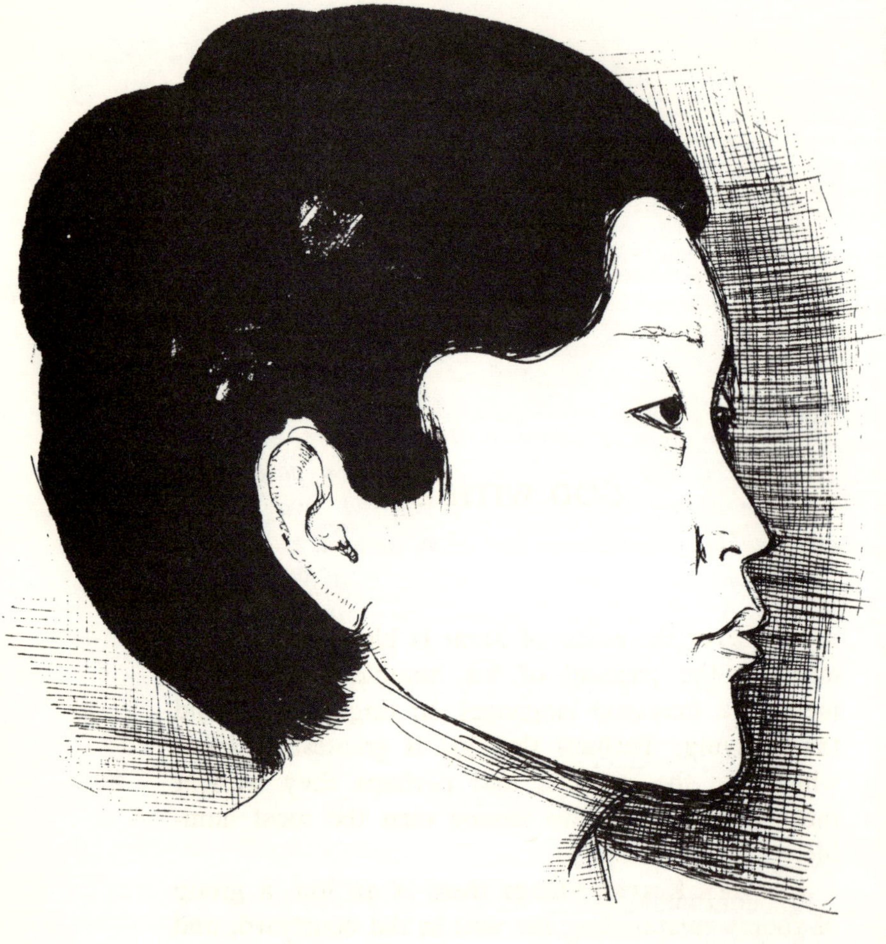

GOD WITH US

Wherever the name of Jesus is blessed at Christmastide, the pageant of his humble birth causes men, in a thousand languages, to sing with joy and thanksgiving. Perhaps that joy is greatest in lands which are the poorest; and perhaps they wonder most whose hearts are among men the most humble.

In every Korean village there is an inn, a group of rooms surrounding the well in the courtyard, and the Oriental visualizes Joseph and Mary beating on the gate seeking shelter, the sleepy innkeeper shouting from within that there is no more room, and thus, to the rice-barn where the rats swarm about, to find shelter and space to lay out a straw mat for a woman in labor. The childbirth, also, quietly dealt with after the manner in which generation after generation of women of the East have borne their children — this too the Koreans understand.

Then came shepherds — but there are no sheep in Korea. Perhaps it was as though a group of farmers, laden with fagots borne on A-frames, descended on a winter's evening from the mountains, there to see in the darkening sky a star such as they'd never before seen; and from the star descending, and brighter than the Milky Way, a dazzling vision of heavenly messengers.

And the wise men. The Korean word is the same as that used for Ph.D.'s: doctors of philosophy from China arriving by palanquin (there's nothing in the Bible about camels) and rendering homage at the rice-shed behind the inn, with a ceremonial bow which brings the forehead to the dust before the King of kings — a newborn babe in the arms of Mary.

So do these humble folk imagine that wondrous story which has become sacred for many of them. The season is devoid of tinsel and sleigh bells, nor are there yule-logs nor holly wreaths nor stockings by a fireplace. A few scraggly pines with roots in earthen pots (for they must be replanted) may be seen in churches and hospitals, decorated with colored paper streamers and cotton balls. That is all. But hours before dawn on Christmas morning, youthful voices may waken you singing, "Glory to

God in the highest, and on earth peace among men with whom he is pleased!" And then you will be reminded that Christmas is a matter of the heart, and that the Christian Korean people, having no wealth, have peace; and receiving few gifts, have yet received the Great Gift. For they know that *God is with us.*

This is the setting for the story of Chung-ja Kang's Christmas gift. At twenty-four years of age her face displayed a rare beauty, and her pensive smile showed elements of hope, fear, trust, and resignation: a Mona Lisa smile on the face of a young wife in whose body lay an unborn child. With her husband she had come to Jesus Hospital seeking relief from the pain of a tumor which was growing in her left shoulder. It was a large mass already causing paralysis of the arm, and our biopsy showed that it was a highly malignant nerve sheath tumor.

We offered her a forequarter amputation — reluctantly, aware that the chances for recurrence were good, yet anxious to save this beautiful girl with the heartrending smile if possible. She and her husband consented. The surgery was done and the tumor cleanly removed and the patient and her husband bravely returned to their home, she having put her trust in Christ, he too bewildered to know what to believe.

A year went by, and they finally heeded our frequent letters begging them to come to Tumor Clinic. It appeared that we had won, that her cancer was controlled, at least temporarily. But one day in the clinic I detected recurrent cancer in her lungs. The baby had died in a distant city after premature childbirth, and now this lovely mother must also walk into the shadows. How tragic her lot! What had she done to deserve this? I could not but wonder as this beautiful Oriental woman probed me with longing eyes: "Am I going to live? Is there hope, doctor?"

Radiation therapy was instituted but was to no avail. The nights lengthened into early winter and her breath became short. Each day on rounds we sought to comfort her, to show her some measure of love. Her husband came and stood by in wretched agony. She read her Bible; she never complained; she moved the hearts of the nurses, the orderlies, the doctors, as she gasped for air and tried to smile.

Shortly before her death, she called the evangelist and said to him, "I will soon die, to go to be with the Lord. I must ask you to do this for me. Please give my Bible to my husband, for he does not yet believe in Jesus, as I believe. And please take this money, just forty cents, it's all I have left — it is not much. Please buy a hymnbook for a beggar-woman." And in a day or two, she was gone. This was shortly after Christmas in the year of our Lord 1963.

A clod was washed away by the sea at a hospital in southwestern Korea. A woman lived her scant twenty-five years and then departed. To what purpose her life? For what her momentary footprint on the sands of time? And yet, two things: The sea that washed away the clod was the ocean of God's mercy. And the other thing — her Christmas gifts. To her beloved husband, her final witness and testament — the Word of God, the source of her peace, the assurance of God's Presence, the basis of her hope in Immanuel. "I have believed. I go in peace. Mayst thou stay in peace. For we have peace with God through our Lord Jesus Christ." And to an unknown beggarwoman, a hymnal. "Believe thou, and praise thou. I know something of suffering: do not fear. Our Lord knows the feelings of our infirmities. He tasted death for every man. He has not failed me. He will not fail you."

Thus did Chung-Ja Kang send her Christmas gifts from her deathbed. To what purpose did she live? Somewhere in Korea a man cherishes the memory of a saint to whom he had the privilege of being married. Her gift to him was the greatest any human being can bestow upon another: the love of God in Christ. Somewhere in Korea a toothless beggar's quavering voice rises uncertainly to sing praises to a Savior. Far more valuable than relief clothing and warm meals received at Jesus Hospital, this worn, dog-eared hymnbook brings back the memory of the gift from one who died victoriously. The husband and the beggar know the meaning of Christmas: God is with us. He gives life; he takes it away; he sends toil and hardship but also love and hope. Throughout all the trials of life he does not abandon me. God is with us.

It is with great hesitation that I would ask you to consider this simple story as part of the answer to the central question in this book, whether God is indeed cognizant of the misery of mankind. Chung-ja Kang's tragedy was of the kind that makes one shake his head, wondering what sense there may be in God's scheme of things, what fairness, what justice, what logic. What answer I may now suggest is not out of any personal experience of suffering.

Dr. Viktor Frankl, the Viennese psychiatrist, has written that human life can be fulfilled not only in creating and enjoying, but also in suffering; that life "can receive its ultimate meaning not only as the result of death, . . . but in the very process of death. Not only the sacrifice of one's life can give meaning; life can reach nobility even as it founders on the rocks."[17] Dr. Frankl is qualified to speak. He experienced the agony of concentration camp existence at Auschwitz. I would not dare suggest that "the right kind of suffering . . . is the highest achievement that has been granted to man."[18] I would not dare suggest this, I say, except for the experience of treating patients like Chung-ja Kang who demonstrated its innate truth. For she attained nobility in her death. She was fully conscious of what was happening. She overcame doubt, self-pity, bitterness, and fear; she accepted God's harsh requirement as she had accepted his loving grace. She not only endured with a faith which was meaningful; she went beyond this. Even when air-hunger made it supremely difficult to speak, she rose to an act of heroic generosity and triumphant testimony. With her final breath she proclaimed her gratitude to Christ.

In God's order of things, death is the condition for life. The life that Jesus lives cannot be revealed in us unless we become like him in his death. Chung-ja Kang carried in her body the death of Jesus: death was at work in her in order that life — the life of Jesus — might be at work in us, who were witnesses to her victory.

The meaning of life is ultimately revealed in the cross of Christ. Apart from Christ, human suffering may be noble, heroic, meaningful, but not finally victorious. With humility I have learned to suggest to those who suffer: "In Christ, your cross may become a resurrection." Human suffering is not only the road to the compassion of God, it is also the pathway to the highest meaning in human existence. The God who transforms curse into blessing also changes death into life.

4

Woe, woe to those who placidly suspire
Drowned in security, remote from fire;
Who under the dim sky and whispering trees
By peaceful slopes and passing streams have ease. . . .
No sacred pang disturbs their secular life,
Eluding splendor and escaping strife;
They die not, for they lived not. . . .
To those whom he doth love God hath not sent
Such dread security, such sad content
But he hath branded on such souls his name,
And he will know them by the scars of flame. . . .
So fear not grief, fear not the anguish, thou,
The paining heart, the clasped and prostrate brow;
This is the emblem, and this is the sign
By which God singles thee for fields divine.[19]

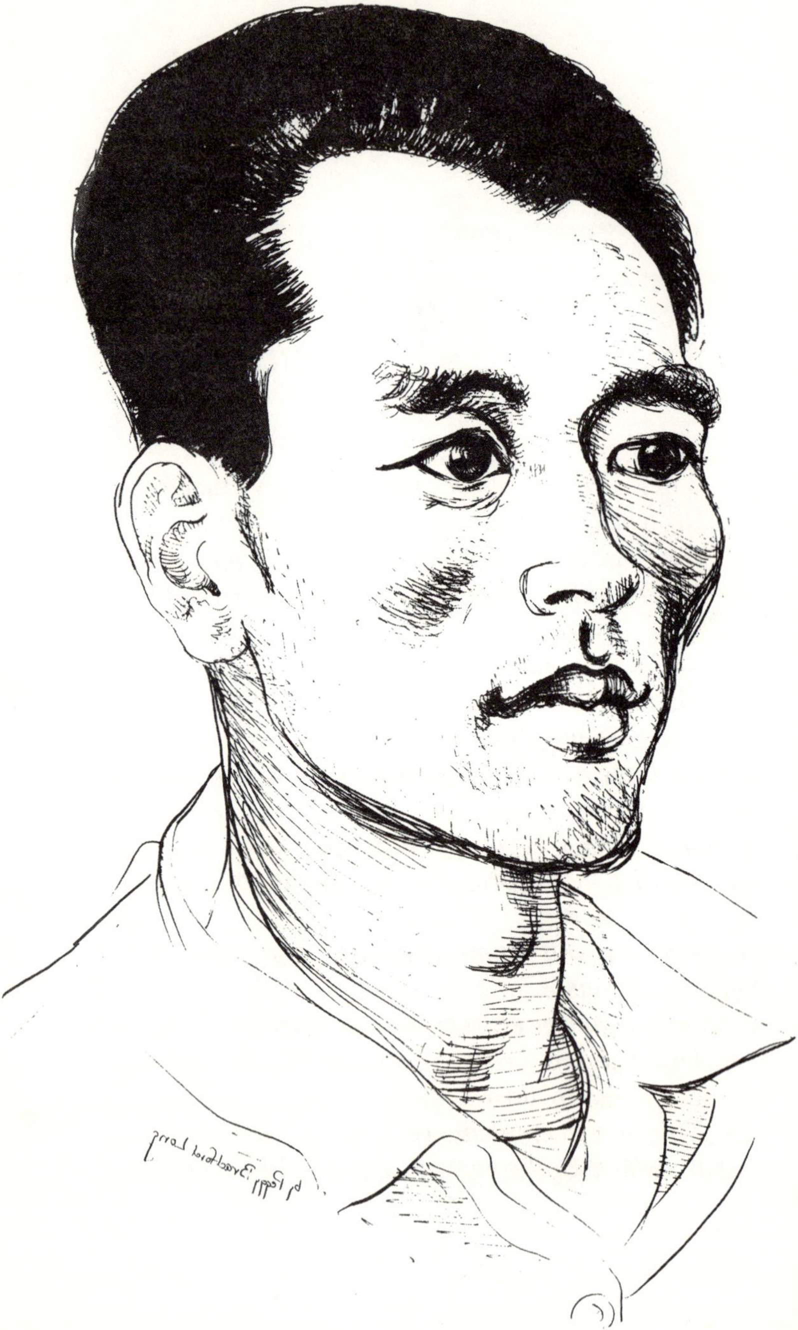

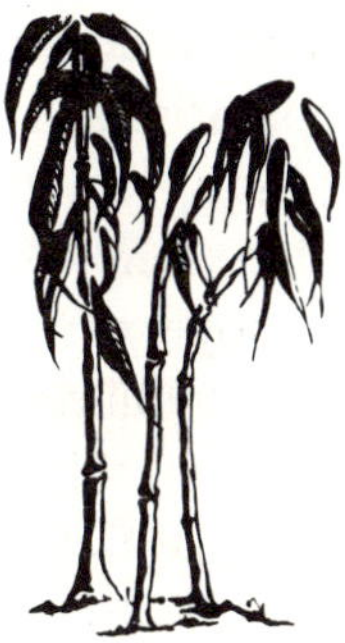

STIGMA

We met him on the way down the hill. He was walking with his crutches, his wife beside him on the way to the bus station. He was pleased to see us, but refused a ride. His wife was more practical. She scurried into the inn where she had been staying, and promptly emerged carrying a bundle wrapped in a scarf, accepting our offer for both of them.

As we rode to the station he did not cease to thank me for his new life. For he was on his way home — home to five children, home to his lodging place (he had lost his house), home to a world of misery and disgrace. For every amputee is disgraced in Korea. Yet he was exultant in his disfigurement, exuberant in his deformity, overjoyed to be alive.

Sang-Hwan Lee had undergone what some would call a mutilating operation, a hemipelvectomy, or hindquarter amputation, to remove an osteosarcoma of the left pelvic bone. He knew that nothing less could offer any hope of curing his cancer. He knew also the bleak possibilities for a destitute, one-legged farmer in Korean society. He did not know, however, that by the very nature of his bone cancer his statistical chance for a cure is a mere ten percent. There are some burdens the cancer surgeon must carry alone — some harsh, inexorable facts, some chilling prognostic expectations.

But the economy of God is not that of man. This cancer business, this interminable parade of misery, protracted death, fatal certainty — how profoundly depressing it is. It would be unbearable without the conviction that the shameful chapter I must witness need not be the end of the story, that despite the bankruptcy of human expectations there is another page in the ledger of eternity for all who accept the legacy of God.

This Sang-Hwan Lee had done. In the discovery of God's love his amputation became somehow unimportant. In the experience of meeting Jesus face to face he found meaning for his life. I do not know whether the joy we witnessed on his homeward journey will survive the chronic dismay which awaits him. I know only that he has embarked upon his own *via crucis,* and that as he hobbles his way up the stony path he will continue to look upward, his gaze fixed on Christ. He does not ask that the stigma be removed, for the stigma and the salvation are for him concomitant, indissoluble, inextricably related.

Is this, perhaps, the way God works in every man?

In the preceding chapter it was suggested that the highest meaning of life is revealed in the cross. The third answer to the basic question under study in this book is related to the second, but is yet distinctive: the *method* of God is also revealed in the cross. If in the story of Chung-ja Kang we came to appreciate the fact that the cross of Christ may give meaning to human suffering, here we go one step beyond: Christ requires participation in his cross. He would suggest that, whether or not every disciple of Jesus is called upon to fulfill the extreme opportunity for triumphant witness, as did Chung-ja Kang, it is probable that every follower of Jesus, without exception, is called to accept his stigma, as did Sang-Hwan Lee. Every one of us must ask himself: Dare we claim the bliss without sharing the pain?

The writer of the epistle to the Hebrews declares:

> Jesus also suffered outside the gate, to consecrate the people by his own blood. Let us then go to him outside the camp, bearing the stigma that he bore.[20]

Let us take a moment to examine this portion of Scripture in its historical and cultural context, for a number of difficulties arise if we apply these words to contemporary society. Where, for example, are the gates of the city in our day? What people are contained within its walls? Where are the boundaries of the camp in our twentieth-century world? Who lies beyond, in the wilderness where Christ died? What is our role toward the homeless, the rejected, the fearful, the disgraced, the forgotten of this world? Who will bear the stigma of Christ?

There have been no walled cities in Western civilization for over a thousand years. In the Orient the walls still stand around many cities, and the gates often serve as monuments to an age whose glory is spent. Therefore the Korean people can well understand their former importance: that the walls served as protection to the citizens in time of danger; that the city government was able to regulate the entry or departure of every person who passed through the gate, and could thus make a distinction between those who belonged and those who did not. Within was security, status, and comfort; outside were the outcasts, the "lepers," the bandits. In ancient Bible times the undesirable elements of society were simply cast out, like refuse. And when a person had committed a crime deserving of death, the execution was carried out outside the city gates, so that the city would not be soiled by the criminal's blood.

Christ was also executed outside the city gates.

His entire life had been a pilgrimage. He had no home of his own. He owned only the clothes he wore. His life was spent among the outcasts and afflicted. And when he gave his life to consecrate these people, this was also beyond the city wall, despised and rejected of men. It was customary that the bodies of animals whose blood was used for a sin-offering by the high priest, were burned outside the camp, "and therefore Jesus also suffered outside the gate,"[21] making of his own body the final disgrace required to atone for the guilt of mankind.

Today the walls are invisible yet often more formidable — barriers of status, prejudice, neglect, apathy, pride. The secure and the affluent enjoy their world of fashion and leisure, shielded from the raw existence of the deprived who vastly outnumber them. In urban America the city has turned inside out. The status holders have captured the perimeter and left a rotting core to the bypassed segment of society. There is no city gate whereby the outcasts might escape the ghetto in which they are trapped.

Yet Christ died in the wilderness; Christ was crucified in the slum; he shed his blood in the distant tribal village, on the remote windswept isle, in the mountain hamlet, beyond the boundaries of the camp. "He had no form or comeliness that we should look at him, . . . and as one from whom men hide their faces he was despised, and we esteemed him not."[22] In a sense, the Suffering Servant yet hangs on the cross beyond the city wall so that God's identification with the despised and the rejected might never be called into question.

Yet the relevance of the Church to the agonies of humanity has been called in question. Can it speak to the wilderness of the world, to the ghetto jungle, to the despondent and disconsolate — until its own heart and soul is branded with the stigma of Jesus?

> Let us then go to him outside the camp,
> bearing the stigma that he bore.

This book in its entirety is concerned with relevance to the human situation. In terms of public health someone may question whether it was worthwhile, the toil and stress of cancer therapy for one of the little ones — the unenlightened, unproductive, forgotten members of the human race. What bearing on human history? What significance in man's quest for the stars? None, save this: here is representative man, the human prototype, the common denominator of mankind, the unit in the mass. Byong-Ho Choi; Chung-ja Kang; Sang-Hwan Lee — these are the unlikely heroes whose experience inspired the account. It has been my privilege to know them, to understand their crisis, their despair, their encounter with Christ, their hesitant, painful, desperate yet victorious walk of faith. The privileged, satiated, transistorized minority "within the city gates" dare not forget the nameless ones beyond the wall. Their very existence may seem as remote as a wave lapping briefly upon some distant shore — until we go to them, and experience the fortitude of their hopes and the pathos of their despair.

We live in a confused age, the more perplexing because mass communications have monopolized our senses, depriving us of the silence necessary to hear the voice of God. His voice is often a cry from the wasteland, what the Koreans call a *si-num-sori,* the sound of groaning of a people longing for deliverance. The Church must hear the sob of grief amid the tumult of technology, the victim's gasping breath beyond the threshhold of abundance.

"Come die with me" — this is the call of Jesus to his people. "Come and join me outside the camp. I have a noose for your head, a gallows for your hanging. Your brand is hot in the fire. The nails are ready for your hands. You must share in my disgrace. If you would be my disciple, you must let me stigmatize your life."

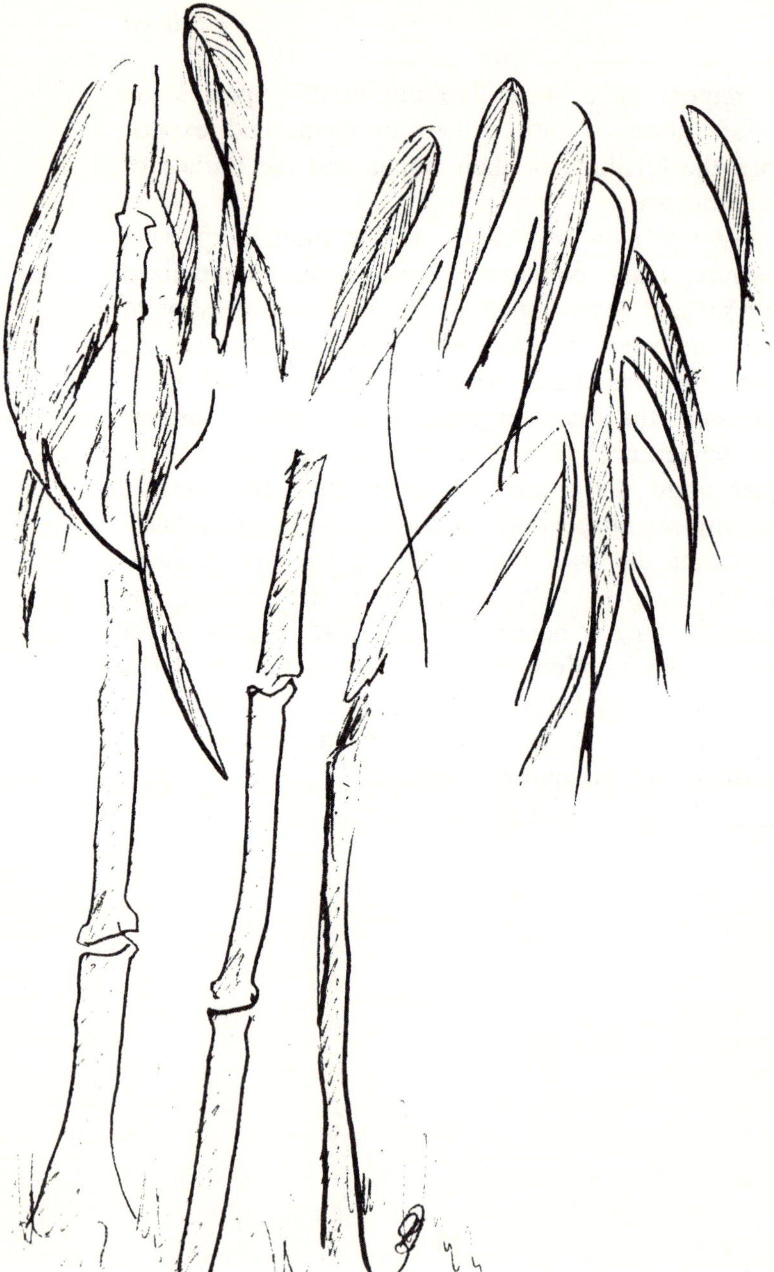

5

"It is not some religious act which makes a Christian what he is, but participation in the sufferings of God in the life of the world."[23]

"The cup of blessing which we bless, is it not a participation in the blood of Christ?"[24]

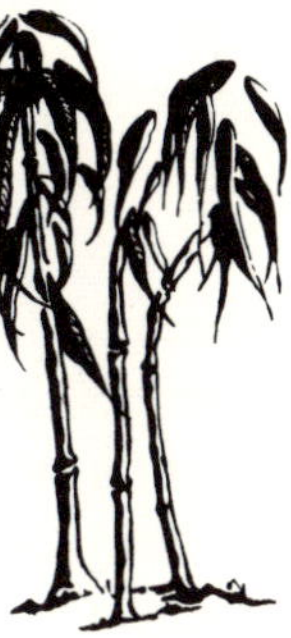

A MEDICAL TESTAMENT

They stood before me in the cold March morning, some in furs, some in farmer's hemp clothing: fifteen survivors of a bloody battle, reassembled now for the celebration. This was Cancer Graduation Day at Jesus Hospital, and these were the graduates. These fifteen, plus thirty more who could not come, were the five-year survivors, all free of disease, from among three hundred cancer patients whom we had attempted to cure in the early 1960s. Each would today receive his diploma:

> This is to certify that Kwak, Young-bae, born in 1914, and afflicted by a malignant tumor, was treated at Jesus Hospital and now in the

> providence of God is free of disease more than five years since treatment.

Mrs. Kwak came forward, received her diploma with both hands, bowed in appreciation, and stepped back.

Looking upon the faces of the group which stood before me in the Quonset chapel that morning, I was transported for fleeting nostalgic moments into a world of battle memories, and felt again the bonds of comradeship in struggle. Here stood Soonduk Kim, the outspoken, devil-may-care, contentious yet courageous woman upon whom I had performed my first anterior exenteration for cancer of the uterine cervix in Korea; well did I recall the tension of that day and her uproarious convalescence. Here also was Byong-Hwan Kang, the schoolteacher, who had almost died from a fulminating lymphoma of the upper jaw, today smiling brightly to show his dental prosthesis. And Mrs. Kwak, whose expressive, rubbery countenance betrayed the conflict of inward thanksgiving and outward propriety. Her chest wall sarcoma had been one of the more vicious-looking enemies I have confronted. One by one they stepped to the podium to receive their graduation certificates. Camera lights flashed, speeches were given, songs of praise were sung. And as I regarded the joy in their faces, the evidence of the faith which had been born in their hearts, I could not but recall the words of Christ:

> . . . If it is by the finger of God that I cast out demons, then the kingdom of God has come upon you.[25]

On more sober reflection I knew that these few from whom the adversary had been cast out were but a small minority of the cancer victims who had come to us. We had saved but one out of six. Our efforts to implement an aggressive thrust in cancer therapy had shown rather limited success. Most had come to us too late. And too many had silent forms of cancer which curtailed their chances further. And I must confess that the catalog of misery which walks before me at Tumor Clinic appalls me even after ten years of cancer work. Is there no end to the charade of life and the parade of death?

Yet I cannot feel regret for having been involved in this uneven contest. It has taught me a profound admiration for contestants whose victories were not always in surviving, but rather in how they failed.

One day in Tumor Clinic, Kum-Dok Noh sat before me, neatly dressed, the large fixed fungating ulcer of the chest wall carefully hidden from sight. Mrs. Noh had had radical surgery for breast cancer elsewhere, and came to us for radiation therapy of recurrent disease. Now she came asking a favor: a diagnostic certificate. It seemed a routine request, until I listened to her. Her husband was in prison, serving a three-year term for burglary. She wanted a document confirming that in a few months she would be dead, in order that her husband might be released to care for her five children.

There were no tears, no pleas for miracle or mercy — only the heroic resignation of someone who in this world has no hope, yet has the courage of her responsibility. She would now take this scrap of paper, this diagnosis of doom, and travel two hundred kilometers to Pusan to besiege the prison fortress where her wayward husband was captive, with her last breath struggling for the survival of her children.

Human tragedy is relative and ubiquitous. Who can understand why catastrophe strikes unexpectedly in natural disasters that destroy hundreds of human lives in a moment? Yet there is a further dimension in the crises of which I speak: these patients have come to Jesus Hospital, have come in effect to the feet of the Savior in their desperation. However much we would rather escape, the weary and heavy-laden have brought their burdens to us. They would risk believing in Christ if it will avail to save their lives. We may most appropriately protest that our God is a God of holiness and righteousness and they must approach him in repentance and seeking forgiveness. We may emphasize that the cross of Christ is effectual for the remission of every man's sin who places his trust in him. But that — in their eyes — is not the issue. They come not with guilt and remorse, but with fear. They seek not salvation but relief from pain. They ask not eternal bliss but a normal life.

The physician's burden, therefore, while offering

health wherever possible, is to open the patient's heart to the greater blessing. We cannot seek to answer his deeper unspoken need unless we first attempt to answer the pain or distress which fills his consciousness. To cure the disease, sometimes; to alleviate suffering, quite often; to extend comfort, always: this is the medical task. But in any event to change the curse into blessing through the power of God: this is the spiritual task.

Heretofore we have not dealt with the specific role of the Christian in the answer to human distress. We have spoken of the *compassion* of God in whose humanity we find comfort, forgiveness, redemption. We have discussed the *significance* of Christ-centered suffering which gives meaning to life. And we have learned that God expects our *participation* in the cross of Christ, that unless we bear his brand he cannot call us his disciples. The first two answers are oriented toward the sufferer. The third is a call to the Christian spectator to leap into the arena, to accept his mark of discipleship. The final proposition, which will be set forth in this and in the subsequent chapter, deals with the relationships which make the disciple effective in uplifting the stricken. *The disciple of Jesus must become involved in God's covenant of mercy.* Christ requires him as an instrument to translate God's mercy into the realm of the sufferer's experience.

In elaborating this thesis we must beg the reader's forbearance. The covenant relationship which we best understand is in the field of medicine. We would here set forth a creed learned at the bedside. It is our anticipation that the same concepts of intelligent assistance, grateful ministry, and intercessory sacrifice will be found applicable in every realm of Christian life. Because it is a covenant relationship we have called this creed a medical testament.

The doctor-patient relationship begins as a commitment of trust. When the physician is also a disciple of Jesus Christ, this commitment is deepened by that disciple's participation in God's purposes. The offer to the patient transcends professional responsibility in all three of its aspects, that of healing, of serving, and of saving.

A Healing Testament

It is a temptation to describe the program at the hospital which is the arena of our struggle: the clinical activities, the teaching emphasis and post-graduate training, the multinational staff of specialists, the teamwork in their common enterprise for Christ, the effort to establish a scientifically competent and evangelically enthusiastic testimony to the glory of our Lord. To describe this endeavor with its ramifications in terms of cost accounting, hospital utilization, free in-patient care, residency program accreditation, statistics of disease incidence, religious requirements for employment, or of mutual benefit agencies for its personnel — would completely frustrate what we are attempting to define.

Rather we must begin quite simply by stating that

in terms of the healing covenant the patient is central. His destiny for a season comes under our jurisdiction. Within our abilities and capabilities no effort is spared to save a life. We have an unusually high proportion of advanced, neglected critically ill patients. Yet we realize in the heat of battle that the cure rate is not the final index of our stewardship.

God speaks to men in events. In a hospital these events are, for practical purposes, the diagnosis and the prognosis of the individual patients. Why did God permit such a deformity, such pain, such misery? Why did he inflict that cancer? Why did he cast the gauntlet of impending death at the feet of some poor, simple, defenseless rice farmer who has never known comfort, has spent his life scrabbling to stay alive and now comes marked for the cauldron? Why? Is it perhaps because God would shake him from the lethargy of his acquiescent complacency, to confront him with the ultimate alternatives of sin and guilt and death, or repentance and trust and life through the cross of Christ? Or is it necessary that in suffering with Christ he shall find meaning for his life?

Healing also is an event of God. In his providence he may grant physical healing, or in his wisdom he may not. In the use of our time, we concentrate primarily on our medical responsibility. Our skills and intellectual powers must be brought captive to Christ as instruments for the accomplishment of his purposes. We recognize no substitute for earnest study or scientific accuracy as far as our responsibility is concerned: in the pursuit of God's truth we dare not test God to compensate for our laziness or intellectual deficiencies. We can testify to the power of prayer in the healing ministry of God; it is the air we breathe, the framework of thought, the substance of our hopes, the fuel in the machinery of decision. Yet it is less than honest to God to expect him to cover by some miraculous intervention the human errors resulting from poor stewardship.

But God's wisdom is inscrutable, and our efforts must ultimately be laid at the feet of Christ: "Lord, we tried, we did our best." And then, at the crux of this ministry, the inescapable question: Did the patient come face to face with Christ? Did he have the option of repentance, the opportunity of responding in gratitude and faith? If not, was it because he did not hear or because he would not listen? Did our concern for him appear so mechanical that his heart was hardened against Jesus, or was his soul filled with gratitude for the measure of Christ's compassion which he experienced?

In the events which break into our lives we must come to recognize the finger of God at work. The event may be great or small, a sudden crisis, or simply an act of kindness. For the patient, the threat of death *is* such an event. God in his mysterious way has plucked a villager from his social milieu, brought him to us, made him vulnerable to the hazard of personal and family catastrophe — for a purpose. God would speak to him: "Listen to me! Listen! The ultimate event in history, the significant event for your life is Christ crucified for your sins. In his body he took your sins to the gallows. By his wounds you may be healed. Trust him. Today is your day of deliverance!"

And so often, in retrospect, we come to see that the byroad was the highway; the interruption in our schedule, the main event; the person, not the disease, the ultimate object; and the healing of his soul at last the only valid cause.

A Serving Testament

God's concern with humanity is expressed in his abasement, whereby he took upon himself the form of a servant. The example of the Great Physician is the guideline of our practice.

There is no higher calling than servanthood. But to interpret this calling into daily action is one of the most difficult tasks of discipleship. Here the distinction between servanthood and service must be made: servanthood requires abasement; service does not. The human spirit does not enjoy abasement. However we may emphasize the concept that carrying bedpans is as honorable as performing delicate surgery, the human instinct for pride and status soon destroys altruistic ideals. True servanthood is perhaps impossible for man except as an act of worship. If the healing testament is patient-centered, the serving testament must be Christ-centered.

We hold sacred the memory of Christ, who washed his disciples' feet. "If I do not wash you, you have no part in me."[26] If Jesus washed our feet, so we ought to wash those of our fellowmen: a servant is not greater than his Master. He even washed the feet of Judas Iscariot. God's abasement to uplift the downtrodden becomes the motivating vision in the hearts of this medical team at the rim of Asia. We would not shrink from the stark realities about us. Rather we must bring Christ into focus in the midst of them: he identified with the hungry, the thirsty, the strangers, the naked, the sick, the imprisoned. We have come to perceive a new significance in human crises:

When rice crop failure portends starvation, it is Jesus, hungry;

When squalor, mendicancy, prostitution, and economic disaster strike our eyes, it is Jesus, a stranger;

When war, refugee camps, orphaned children — the spectacle of urchins huddled under newspaper in winter — disturb us, it is Jesus, naked;

When illness and suffering strike, when the deathmakers and life-cripplers of a helpless society cast their victims upon our threshhold, we recognize in the form of the afflicted, Christ, our patient;

When prison walls, concentration camps, economic enslavement and racial prejudice fetter any human being, it is Christ, in prison.

Christ puts himself in their place. He champions the downtrodden, the refuse of this inhuman planet. He honors every fragment of the human race, however miserable, however foul, for he tells us that if we would serve him, we must serve them; if we would glorify him, we must honor them. "Inasmuch as ye have done it unto one of the least of these my brethren, ye have done it unto me."[27]

Christ puts himself in their skin, takes upon himself their ulcers, their cancers, their festering wounds. The medical disciple of Jesus has the privilege of looking upon every anguished soul and remembering that Christ lies there: Christ, my patient — his the pain, his the stench, the shame, the despair.

We have come to understand the meaning of Christ's plea. The highest expression of devotion to our Lord will be found in sacrificial ministry toward those whom he honors by his love. If we would bring an offering of gratitude, if we would anoint Jesus with our worship, we must anoint the wounds of body and of spirit of the afflicted whom Christ sends in his stead. This is the serving testament.

A Saving Testament

In the healing ministry, the patient is central. He becomes the highest cause. Christ is focusing his mercy through us upon him. In the serving ministry, Christ is central. To anoint those with whose human frailty he identifies becomes the noblest worship; we are focusing our gratitude upon Christ through the patient. In the saving ministry, the Cross is central. It is become the focus of God's holiness, love, mercy, and righteousness in dealing with the entire human race.

In the final analysis, the Christian's covenant is his participation in the death of Christ. This is not to suggest in any sense a dilution of, or infringement upon, the messiahship of Jesus, upon the sufficiency of his cross in the expiation of human sin, upon the uniqueness of the divine intervention for man by the Son of God, or upon the sovereignty of Christ in reconciling all men unto himself through the blood of the cross.

The cross which Christ requires his disciples to lift is voluntary yet essential. It may be possible to be a Christian without carrying it; it is not possible to be a disciple without carrying it. For those who choose to be crucified with Christ there is a mystery of participation in his redemptive work: we may become the framework for the power of the cross of our Lord to become fully operative toward some individual. Paul referred to completing, in his flesh, "what is lacking in Christ's afflictions."[28]

Obviously, from the perspective of the *effectiveness* of Christ's sacrifice, if God was satisfied by the travail of his soul in expiating the full weight of the world's sin, how can Paul or anyone else "complete what is lacking" in Christ's sufferings? Yet from the perspective of the *application* of Christ's sacrifice to the unsaved human conscience, is it unreasonable, is it not rather imperative, that the disciple participate in the cross? "The cup of blessing which we bless, is it not participation in the blood of Christ?"

Every blessing we would render has a price. We are not called to a cheap charity. The care of the cancer patient requires the sacrifice of time, energy, and concern. In dissecting out a cancer, six, seven, eight, or more hours of effort may be expended. The dedication of time and energy and concern is what makes credible our medical testament to the saving love of Christ. Whoever would know Christ and experience the power of his resurrection must also share in his suffering, in growing conformity to his death.

There is nothing unique in, or conditional to, the medical Christian experience in the expression of the mercy covenant of God which we have outlined. Healing, serving, saving, and loving: all are essential in the interpretation of God's concern at the level of the extreme experiences of life. In the last chapter we will seek to take the covenant relationship to its highest expression as we explore the dynamism of Christ-centered bonds of love.

The Latin phrase *via crucis* actually encompasses much of what we have been trying to express throughout the book. It was the heart of Isaiah's prophecy, the central fact of Jesus' life. It is the process of our salvation, the truth which gives meaning to suffering, the requirement for Christian discipleship, and the means for the expression of God's mercy to our fellowmen, particularly to those who suffer. The way of the cross is nowhere better described than in the words of Paul the apostle: "We are afflicted in every way, but not crushed; perplexed, but not driven to despair; persecuted, but not forsaken; struck down, but not destroyed; always carrying in the body the death of Jesus, so that the life of Jesus may also be manifested in our bodies."[29]

6

What makes loneliness an anguish
Is not that I have no one to share my burden,
But this:
I have only my own burden to bear. . . .
Pray that your loneliness may spur you into finding something to live for, great enough to die for.[30]

To love life and men as God loves them — for the sake of their infinite possibilities.[31]

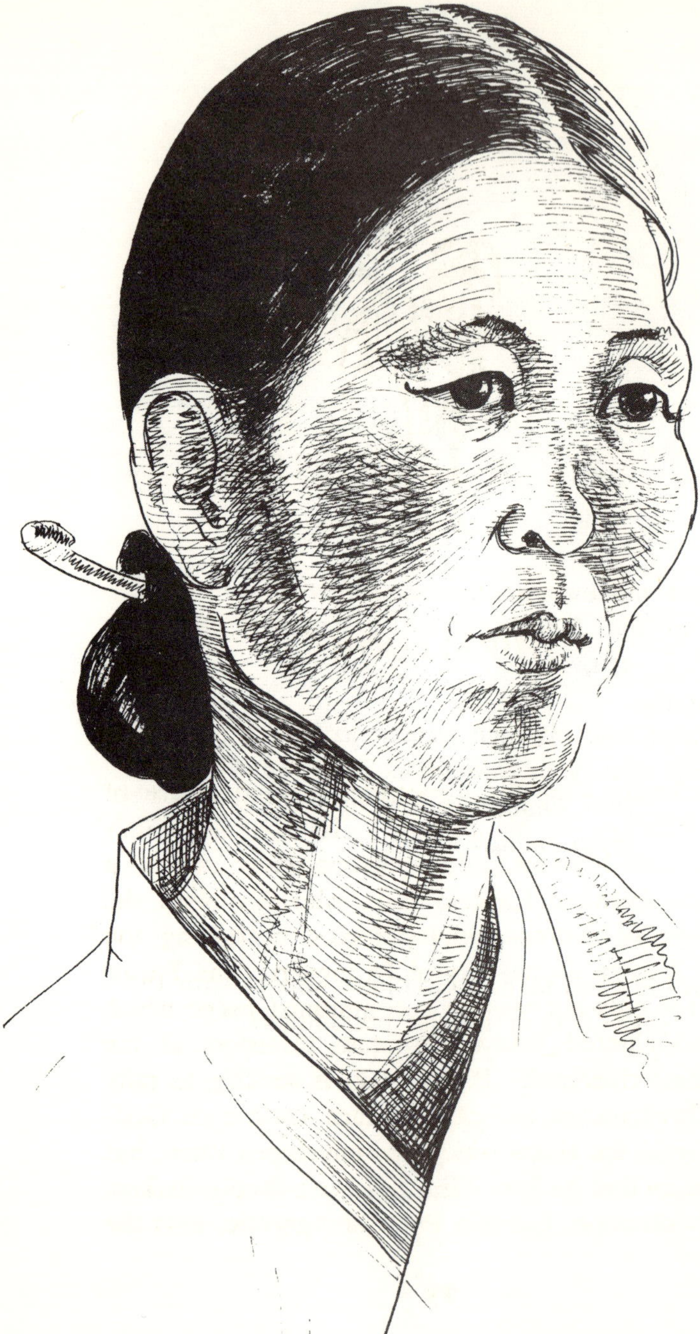

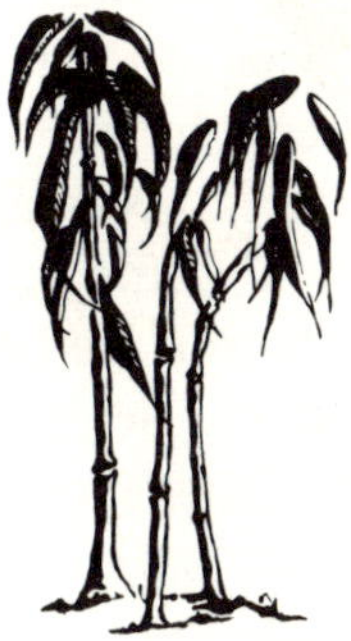

THRALLDOM

We began with the question, "Is God aware of the sufferings of his people?" In Richard Kim's novel, *The Martyred,* the question grew out of a dialogue between Captain Pak, who was with the Republic of Korea military forces occupying the North Korean capital city of Pyongyang, and Pastor Shin, the only survivor of a communist purge which had slaughtered twelve Christian ministers at the Tae-dong riverbank. Pastor Shin is seeking to rally the Christians in the city, to turn their eyes Godward amid the chaos which has enveloped them, but it appears that his own faith has been deeply shaken. In this situation, Captain Pak, the agnostic, puts the question which reveals the doubt in the heart of the minister of God.

An uneasy peace prevails in Korea today, and the question has been refocused upon a more personal form of chaos. In order to make the inquiry a meaningful one it is necessary to bring it to bear upon mankind in a comparable pit of desolation and misery. The cancer victim would appear to be a valid case in point. Seldom is man apt to feel more helpless physically, more bankrupt psychologically, than when he harbors, and knows that he harbors, an enemy within which would destroy him. The situation becomes all the more precarious when his economic resources are virtually nonexistent, and when his cultural and religious heritage makes him alien to the concept of a personal God.

In this book we have attempted an honest answer to a question which cannot be lightly dismissed. The Scriptures indeed speak to this situation, as they did to Job and to the Babylonian exiles and to the cripple on Solomon's Porch. To the wretched and miserable, God says: "The bruised reed I will not break; the smoldering wick I will not quench. You are precious in my eyes, and honored, and I love you." Yet it becomes difficult to accept God's words at face value unless they are the words of a God who became man, who not only knows the human predicament but humbled himself beyond the bottom level of human existence. This Jesus was subjected to the trauma of life, died afflicted by the spiritual cancers of the world, descended into hell, was raised from the dead, and lives today. Each clause in the statement is necessary if we would have a case for hope.

Yet this answer, and all of the answers God reveals to his own people, must be proclaimed. The cross of compassion, the cross of significance, the cross of participation — the very soul of the yearning God may not become relevant or applicable to the distress of one individual without the cross of covenant. The reality of the humanity of God must be poured into the existential flask where every man is tested; and for this task God generally requires the obedient service of those who know him, the redeemed becoming participants in the redemptive endeavor.

In this chapter we would examine more deeply the nature of the redemptive relationship.

We have just set forth, in Chapter 5, a philosophy of Christian medical responsibility which we have designated a medical *testament*. By the use of this word we have sought to indicate a contract relationship which, when offered up to God, may become dynamic. We offer this to the reader as an experimental model for human intercourse under God the Father, knowing full well that it is idealistic, and practicable only in varying degrees, yet believing that it is valid in all horizontal relationships in the family of man. Once again we employ the doctor-patient relationship as a framework for our discussion.

We would briefly review some of the concepts of

responsibility and concern which have broad acceptance in the field of medical ethics today. Although the altruism of the medical profession has become tarnished in the eyes of a public which expects more of the physician than it expects of itself, it remains generally true that doctors are motivated, at least in part, by noble ideals in their role as guardians of physical life. Nevertheless, there are different views as to how this responsibility must be carried in regard to the "whole man."

Sir William Osler was professor of medicine at the University of Pennsylvania from 1884 until 1889, and at Johns Hopkins until 1905. For over twenty years he served as one of the truly great teachers and clinicians in medical history. In his valedictory address at the University of Pennsylvania, he counseled his students and colleagues to cultivate imperturbability and equanimity under all circumstances. It was a courageous creed in a difficult time, before typhoid, yellow fever, and tuberculosis had been brought under control, a day in which physicians often felt themselves to be little more than "useful supernumeraries in the battle, . . . stage accessories in the drama, playing minor, but essential, parts in the exits or entrances, or picking up, here and there, a strutter who may have tripped upon the stage." Speaking to a class of graduating nurses in 1891, he went on to say, "You have been much by the dark river . . . and have seen so many embark, that the dread of the old boatman has almost disappeared. . . . Your (own) passport shall be the blessing of Him in whose footsteps you have trodden, unto whose sick you have ministered, and for whose children you have cared."[32] It is hard to imagine a more noble propriety, a kindness couched in greater dignity.

Osler's call for equanimity in the storm of crisis has been echoed in the marble halls of medicine throughout the world. His was an appeal for detachment in order to allow the physician to render objective judgment, and make possible cool decisiveness in professional life: "Cultivate, then, gentlemen, such a judicious measure of obtuseness as will enable you to meet the exigencies of practice with firmness and courage without, at the same time, 'hardening the heart by which we live.' "[33] Sir William's guiding principle, *aequanimitas,* might thus be termed "kindly detachment"; it is reflected in the feelings of most physicians today that propriety precludes involvement in the spiritual dimensions of a patient's problems.

A more idealistic formula was embodied in the life of the great humanitarian of Lambaréné, Dr. Albert Schweitzer. The three pillars of motivation upon which he built his hospital in equatorial Africa were "the Fellowship of those who bear the Mark of Pain," the moral obligation of the European towards the natives of Central Africa, and the ethic of reverence for life. His biographer, Werner Picht, states that few could support him in the first two ideological concepts. The third, on the other hand, electrified the world and caused his name to become a byword for the highest ethical aspirations of man.

In discussing Dr. Schweitzer's thought we are concerned here only with the doctor-patient relationship; his theological position does not have direct bearing upon the discussion. His act of renunciation in committing himself to the service of mankind in the jungle gave moral force to his ethical convictions. Yet it remains a question whether he was capable of fraternal love toward his African patients, a love which sought the fulfillment of their potential. He was obsessed by the vision of noble sacrifice, the obligation of atonement, the sanctity of all forms of physical life — human or animal — and it appears that the personhood of his patient was lost. To quote his biographer:

> The way of "reverence for life" adopted by Schweitzer does not culminate in the loving care for the individual and his well-being, but in the general struggle against pain and disease. His contact with the Negroes is brought about by physical crises in their lives and it usually ends when they have been overcome, so that generally speaking it is impossible to exercise a profounder influence upon them. The struggle against pain is carried on in an unending series of individual acts, and this form of charity is in complete accordance with the will ethic of Schweitzer. It demands service to threatened life and not to any individual personality. This springs from its equalization of all forms of life. With compelling logic therefore human life appears as something anonymous. The apostle of rev-

> erence for life has to bear the burden of working as a human being amongst human beings who pass before him as unknowns in a horrible procession of innocent sufferers from the self-alienation of life, hoping always that he can alleviate their pain and suffering.[34]

In recent years a third concept of doctor-patient responsibility has been set forth by the brilliant Viennese psychiatrist, Dr. Viktor Frankl, the proponent of the new field of logotherapy and existential analysis. Out of his own concentration camp experience he elaborated the concept of will-to-meaning, the basic need for the human psyche to have a goal in life. As a practicing psychiatrist, Frankl has crossed the great divide between psyche and spirit. He maintains that medicine must operate along this great divide, this no-man's land, in order to help individuals to attain their potentialities and find meaning in their suffering.

All three, Osler, Schweitzer, and Frankl, acknowledged God. Their views of the role of the medical profession in doctor-patient relationships vary. Osler's *noble detachment* reflects his convictions that spiritual matters are beyond his jurisdiction. Schweitzer's *reverence for life* may have become an obstacle in seeing the patient as a person to be loved. Frankl's *medical ministry* affirms the uniqueness of the individual; he would risk entering the realm of the spirit (which Osler would not), and recognizes the need of every person for a purpose (which Schweitzer evaded). Yet Frankl falls short of proclaiming any fixed point of reference in the search for value worthy of commitment:

> Existential analysis remains non-committal on the question of "to what" a person should feel responsible — whether to his God or his society or his conscience or whatever higher power. And existential analysis equally forbears to say what a person should feel responsible for — for the realization of which values, for the fulfillment of which personal tasks, for which particular meaning to life.[35]

Noble concepts, all three. None adequate for a medical disciple of Jesus Christ. In fairness, at least two of them were not intended to be. It remains necessary then to define the doctor-patient relationship in the framework of the Christian faith, for this has ever been a healing faith. Jesus healed and commanded to heal. His orders were taken literally by his apostles, beginning with the healing by Peter and John of the lame man at the gate called Beautiful. During the early centuries of the middle ages, convents and monasteries became centers of medical care. St. Benedict told his monks: "The care of the sick is to be attended to before all things."[36] In recent times also churches have felt a responsibility for establishing hospitals and medical centers in the homeland, and medical outposts abroad. With the increasing complexity of medical science most church-related institutions have outgrown the religious framework, and the churches have turned over to government or private control their noble ventures. The author knows of four medical schools around the world, of Protestant tradition, which remain Christian in terms of commitment to honor Christ primarily. The ministry of healing in the name of Jesus devolves almost entirely upon the practicing Christian physician, supported abroad by the medical missionary thrust.

Yet as never before the proclamation of the mercy of God requires participation in God's mercy. God is aware of the sufferings of his people. The question is, *are we?* Christ calls upon us to do something about it, to proclaim his love, his concern, his holiness, his cross, his forgiveness, his redemption, his healing. Almost in one breath he says to the paralytic: "Your sins are forgiven you. . . . Rise and walk." How may we translate his total ministry into the practical requirements of this century?

The redemptive relationship of which we speak is not accomplished with human resources. The contract of which we speak is neither direct nor reciprocal, but *triangular.* Christ reaches down to the person through his disciple. The disciple worships Christ through the person. And in the experience, *both* the disciple and the person (i.e., doctor and patient, businessman and associate, housewife and neighbor, professor and colleague, farmer and friend) *come under the Cross.*

In the covenant of healing, the flow of energy is from Christ through the physician (instrument) to the patient (focus). In the covenant of serving, the flow of energy is from the doctor through the patient (instrument) to Christ (focus). In the covenant of salvation, the flow is from Christ through his cross (instrument) toward mankind (focus).

The equanimity which Osler sought is realized not by detachment but by involvement on behalf of Christ. The physician, free from dependence upon the limits imposed by his own resources, looks to God for power and commits to God for inner peace. The reverence for life which Schweitzer sought is realized not as some idealistic concept but is fulfilled in the act of anointing the patient whom Christ sent in his stead; in worshiping Christ who is the source of life. The pursuit of meaning for life which Frankl sought becomes a reality when the patient apprehends the meaning of Christ: that he is the object of Christ's love, and that through his cross he may be forgiven.

But doctor-patient relationships have been discussed simply as illustrations of any interpersonal relationship in which two persons (at least one of them a disciple of Christ) come to grips with a problem of human distress. What we speak of here might be called intercessory discipleship. It stems from the deepest yearnings of the soul to be used, to show gratitude, to "become." Or, as Dag Hammarskjöld phrased it, "to love life and men as God loves them — for the sake of their infinite possibilities."

If life is indeed to achieve its fullest meaning, every person must find his unique destiny and become aware of the divine blueprint for his life. For the disciple of Jesus this requires *being used* by God for one's fellowman. If life is to have its fullest meaning, every person must find a cause to worship, "something to live for, great enough to die for." For the follower of Jesus this requires a tangible, pragmatic means of *showing* the *gratitude* he feels toward his Savior. If life is indeed to have its fullest meaning, each man must find a means for growth and renewal. For the disciple of Jesus this is fulfilled in God's promise that whoever believes in Christ is granted power *to become* a child of God.

We began with a two-dimension doctor-patient contract; we have returned now to a three-dimensional interpersonal covenant. We began with the necessity of participating in God's mercy out of concern for the sufferings of God's people; we conclude with a participation in God's mercy to fulfill the deepest longings of our souls. We began bound to Christ by obedience and gratitude and to our fellowman in altruistic effort; we conclude bound to Christ and to our fellowman in the thralldom of his love. What happened? When the relationship was brought to the foot of the Cross, Christ entered into it and transformed it. It now bears the stamp of his grace.

In closing, I have searched for an illustration which might, in however pale and fragmentary a manner, speak of the covenant of love. In my experience it has been fleeting but real, easily lost in the hurly-burly of medical practice, yet more to be cherished than any other experience in the clinical realm or any other realm of human contact. Such is the kinship I have felt toward Ho-Yul Lee.

She came to us in 1963, a widow of forty-five, with a huge cancer of the thyroid gland, presenting as a mass on the right neck which was as large as her head, ulcerating and bleeding. For seventeen years this tumor had grown fatter and sleeker at her expense, and she came at last in what appeared to be a hopeless situation. However, there was no evidence of metastasis, and we decided to risk a surgical attack. A large preliminary skin flap was outlined to allow covering of the tumor site. Radical neck dissection was then performed, sacrificing the clavicle to allow purchase on the jugular vein at its origin at the thoracic inlet. It was a gamble: it was impossible to tell whether the carotid artery was involved prior to resection. Fortunately the tumor came off clean. Her post-operative course was difficult but eventually she went home free of disease. For two years she attended Tumor Clinic — then silence. Our follow-up letters were returned undelivered.

More than five years after her surgery I ventured out to find her on a mountain plateau seventy-five miles from Chonju. This highland is located within the Chiri mountain range, but north of the peaks. My wife, Mary, accompanied me. We drove the Land Cruiser off the county road, along a narrow byway to the precinct office by a spreading oak. From here we were directed along an ox-cart path across several fords to the village of Akokni, a hamlet of fifty or sixty houses at the edge of nowhere. When the road ended, we proceeded on foot and were met by a swarm of children. Eventually several women met us, and we asked for Mrs. Ho-Yul Lee. No one recognized the name. Nonplussed, we explained why we had come — to find a lady who years ago had undergone surgery for a huge tumor of the neck.

"Oh, you mean Tok-tong Taek!"

This was, then, her nickname in town, we surmised. We followed the women into the thatched-roof hamlet, through narrow alleys between mud walls, followed by the inevitable procession of youngsters. The village ended. Beyond it we found a smaller dwelling on the hillside at the end of the path: two rooms, one of them an earth-floor kitchen, one a hot-floor room eight by eight feet, with tattered paper door, padlocked. Her ten-year-old daughter playing in the brook nearby volunteered to find her, for she was in the paddy fields, transplanting rice. She came presently, the same staunch, frail figure I remembered so well, her face ordinary but radiant, a bouquet of daisies in the sun. Her voice was hoarse — we had sacrificed one of the nerves to her vocal cords — but she spoke clearly, fervently, "Oh, doctor, I am grateful!"

There is not much more to the story. We talked and laughed with her and with most of the women in the community. Mrs. Lee had become a Christian five years before, but this was the first effort anyone had made to bring her to the church, or bring the church to her. She was illiterate, virtually nameless, almost homeless. She could only whisper; the cancer had left its mark, the cure was survived by its stigma. But Christ knew her; and she remembered Christ. Into her small, meaningless life a light had shined, the slender ray of the sun penetrating a dark forest.

Christ himself was present at our meeting. He transformed the moment. Mary, standing beside me, felt also the bonds of fellowship towards this frail figure at the end of the world, with whom we had established a covenant which held us in thrall.

Notes

Preface

1. Richard E. Kim, *The Martyred* (Seoul, Korea: Sam Jung Dang), p. 37. Used by permission.

Chapter 1

2. William Faulkner, *Requiem for a Nun* (New York: New American Library of World Literature, 1961). Used by permission.
3. Isaiah 43:1-3 (RSV).
4. Isaiah 42:1-4 (RSV).
5. Luke 4:18, 19 (from Isaiah 61:1, 2; RSV).
6. John 3:16 (KJV).
7. John 14:18 (RSV).

CHAPTER 2

8. Richard C. Lippincott, "The Physician's Approach to Cancer," *Surgical Clinics of North America* 47:3:559, June 1967. Used by permission.
9. Job 19:25, 26 (KJV).
10. Hugh J. Mooney, "What the Cigarette Commercials Don't Show," *Christian Herald,* October, 1967. Used by permission.
11. Ethelwyn Wetherald, "My Orders."
12. 1 Corinthians 9:16 (KJV).
13. Romans 3:13-18 (KJV).
14. Romans 7:24 (KJV).

CHAPTER 3

15. John Donne, "Devotions XVII," *The Complete Poetry and Selected Prose of John Donne, and the Complete Poetry of William Blake* (New York: Random House, 1946), *The Modern Library.* Used by permission.
16. 2 Corinthians 4:11, 12 (NEB).
17. Viktor Frankl, *The Doctor and the Soul* (New York: Bantam Books, 1967), p. 85. Used by permission.
18. Ibid., Introduction, p. xii.

CHAPTER 4

19. Stephen Phillips, "Grief and God," (London: The Bodley Head, 1930). Used by permission.
20. Hebrews 13:12, 13 (NEB).
21. Ibid.
22. Isaiah 53:2, 3 (RSV).

CHAPTER 5

23. Dietrich Bonhoeffer, *Letters and Papers from Prison* (New York: Macmillan Company, 1953), p. 223. Used by permission.
24. 1 Corinthians 10:16 (RSV).
25. Luke 11:20 (RSV).
26. John 13:8 (RSV).
27. Matthew 25:40 (KJV).
28. Colossians 1:24 (KJV).
29. 2 Corinthians 4:8-10 (RSV).

CHAPTER 6

30. Dag Hammarskjöld, *Markings* (New York: Alfred A. Knopf, 1965), p. 85. Used by permission.
31. Ibid., p. 127.
32. William Osler, *Aequanimitas with Other Addresses to Medical Students, Nurses and Practitioners of Medicine* (Philadelphia, P. Blakiston and Sons, 1932), p. 19. Used with permission of McGraw-Hill Book Company.
33. Ibid., p. 5.
34. Werner Picht, *The Life and Thought of Albert Schweitzer* (New York: Harper and Row, 1964), p. 153. Used by permission.
35. Viktor Frankl, Op. cit., p. 224.
36. Louis Lasagna, *The Doctor's Dilemma* (New York: Harper and Bros., 1962), p. 81. Used by permission.

Glossary

Page	
14	*carcinogenic:* Causing or producing cancer. A carcinogen is any substance which causes cancer.
21	*septicemia:* An infection of the blood stream; a condition due to presence of disease-forming organisms and associated poisons in the blood.
28	*lesion:* Any hurt, wound, degeneration, or tumor. The term "primary lesions" refers generally to new growths from specific sites.
29	*uterine cervix:* The narrow lower end of the uterus.
30	*oncology:* Sum knowledge regarding tumors or new growths.
35	*biopsy:* Examination of tissue removed from a living subject. In popular usage, a biopsy may be said to be positive or negative depending on the presence or absence of cancer cells in the tissue examined.

Does My Father Know I'm Hurt?

45 *forequarter amputation:* Amputation of the upper extremity (arm) and shoulder girdle, including shoulder blade and collar bone.

54 *hemipelvectomy:* Amputation of the lower extremity (leg) and half of the pelvis, i.e., "hipbone."

54 *prognostic:* Related to the prediction of the probable result of disease.

64 *anterior exenteration:* The radical removal of the anterior organs of the pelvic cavity (all organs except the rectum) for cancer.

64 *lymphoma:* A family of cancer that usually arise in the lymph nodes, but may also originate in lymphatic or specialized lining cells in other organs.

64 *prosthesis:* An artificial organ (as an eye, leg, or denture) which serves as a replacement for an absent part.

64 *sarcoma:* A cancer of supporting tissues (as compared with *carcinoma,* which is a cancer of lining or glandular tissues).

90 *metastasis:* Transfer of disease from one organ to another. Commonly used in regard to cancer spread from the primary site to another organ by means of the blood or lymphatic circulation.

90 *radical neck dissection:* Radical removal of all lymph node-bearing areas in the neck including the jugular vein and certain muscles.

90 *clavicle:* "collarbone."